Remedy For Blood Disease In Men

A Complete Guide To Managing Blood Disorder

by

John J. Smith

Table of content

INTRODUCTION

Your blood is a living tissue composed of fluid and solids. The liquid part, called plasma, is made of water, salts, and protein. Over a portion of your blood is plasma. The strong aspect of your blood contains red platelets, white platelets, and platelets.

Blood issues influence at least one piece of the blood and keep your blood from taking care of its business. They can be intense or constant. Many blood issues are acquired. Different causes incorporate different sicknesses, symptoms of drugs, and an absence of specific supplements in your eating routine.

The area of hematology envelops a wide exhibit of conditions influencing the blood, and progressions in clinical science have prompted imaginative answers for different blood issues. From problems of coagulating and draining to irregularities in red and white platelets, specialists and medical services experts constantly endeavor to foster compelling therapies. This presentation digs into the different scenes of answers for blood issues, investigating advancement treatments, hereditary mediations, and developing clinical advances that hold guarantee in working on the anticipation and personal satisfaction of people wrestling with hematological difficulties.

Blood issues include a different cluster of ailments that influence the structure, capability, or creation of blood parts inside the human body. From acquired hereditary issues to acquired conditions, blood problems present huge difficulties to well-being and prosperity. As how we might interpret hematological circumstances propels, so too does the journey for compelling answers to address these intricate difficulties.

In recent years, advancements in clinical examination and innovation have prompted a more profound cognizance of the fundamental systems driving different blood issues. This uplifted comprehension has prepared for inventive and designated helpful intercessions. The journey for answers to blood issues includes a multidisciplinary approach, uniting hematologists, geneticists, pharmacologists, and other clinical experts to foster thorough procedures that address the remarkable qualities of each problem.

One of the basic support points in the treatment of blood problems is pharmacotherapy. Drugs intended to tweak platelet creation, improve coagulation factors, or smother strangely resistant reactions assume a focal role in overseeing numerous hematological circumstances.

From anticoagulants that forestall blood clump arrangement to development factors that animate red platelet creation, drug mediations mean to reestablish the sensitive equilibrium inside the circulation system.

Blood bondings address one more foundation for tending to blood issues. For conditions portrayed by lacking or failing blood parts, for example, pallor or certain coagulation problems, bondings provide fundamental donor blood that, painstakingly screened and matched to the beneficiary, can renew drained components and further develop general blood capability. Notwithstanding, the maintainability and accessibility of contributor blood remain continuous difficulties that analysts and medical care suppliers keep on tending to.

In situations where hereditary elements contribute to blood problems, state-of-the-art improvements in quality treatment offer promising roads for treatment. The capacity to change or supplant broken qualities opens additional opportunities for tending to the underlying drivers of acquired blood problems. As exploration in this field advances, the potential for customized and corrective methodologies turns out to be progressively unmistakable.

Past these traditional strategies and rising advancements, for example, CRISPR-Cas9 quality altering holds groundbreaking possibilities in the domain of blood problem arrangements. The capacity to definitively alter hereditary material raises moral contemplations yet additionally opens ways to adjust hereditary irregularities at their source. The excursion toward saddling the full force of quality alteration with regard to blood problems is one of both fervor and cautious moral consultation.

Notwithstanding clinical mediations, way-of-life adjustments and steady consideration assume essential parts in overseeing blood issues. Dietary changes, actual work, and stress on the board contribute to general prosperity and can supplement clinical medicines. Schooling and support for people with blood problems and their families are fundamental parts of a complete methodology, cultivating strengthening and flexibility notwithstanding ongoing circumstances.

Cooperation between specialists, medical services suppliers, and promotion bunches is fundamental to driving advancement in the field of blood problem arrangements. By cultivating an aggregate comprehension of the difficulties presented by these circumstances, partners can cooperate to upgrade findings, further develop treatment choices, and eventually lift the personal satisfaction of people impacted by blood problems.

All in all, the scene of blood problem arrangements is developing quickly, pushed by logical forward leaps, mechanical developments, and a cooperative obligation to propel patient consideration. This presentation gives a brief look into the complex methodologies utilized to address blood problems, underscoring the continuous quest for extensive, customized, and morally sound arrangements that guarantee to reclassify the fate of hematological medication.

Your blood is a living tissue composed of fluid and solids. The liquid part, called plasma, is made of water, salts, and protein. Over a portion of your blood is plasma. The strong aspect of your blood contains red platelets, white platelets, and platelets.

Blood issues influence at least one piece of the blood and keep your blood from taking care of its business. They can be intense or constant. Many blood issues are acquired.

Different causes incorporate different sicknesses, symptoms of drugs, and an absence of specific supplements in your eating routine.

The area of hematology envelops a wide exhibit of conditions influencing the blood, and progressions in clinical science have prompted imaginative answers for different blood issues. From problems of coagulating and draining to irregularities in red and white platelets, specialists and medical services experts constantly endeavor to foster compelling therapies. This presentation digs into the different scenes of answers for blood issues, investigating advancement treatments, hereditary mediations, and developing clinical advances that hold guarantee in working on the anticipation and personal satisfaction of people wrestling with hematological difficulties.

Blood issues include a different cluster of ailments that influence the structure, capability, or creation of blood parts inside the human body. From acquired hereditary issues to acquired conditions, blood problems present huge difficulties to well-being and prosperity. As how we might interpret hematological circumstances propels, so too does the journey for compelling answers to address these intricate difficulties.

In recent years, advancements in clinical examination and innovation have prompted a more profound cognizance of the fundamental systems driving different blood issues. This uplifted comprehension has prepared for inventive and designated helpful intercessions. The journey for answers to blood issues includes a multidisciplinary approach, uniting hematologists, geneticists, pharmacologists, and other clinical experts to foster thorough procedures that address the remarkable qualities of each problem.

One of the basic support points in the treatment of blood problems is pharmacotherapy. Drugs intended to tweak platelet creation, improve coagulation factors, or smother strangely resistant reactions assume a focal role in overseeing numerous hematological circumstances. From anticoagulants that forestall blood clump arrangement to development factors that animate red platelet creation, drug mediations mean to reestablish the sensitive equilibrium inside the circulation system.

Blood bondings address one more foundation for tending to blood issues. For conditions portrayed by lacking or failing blood parts, for example, pallor or certain coagulation problems, bondings provide fundamental help. Giving blood, painstakingly screened and matched to the beneficiary, can renew drained components and further develop general blood capability. Notwithstanding, the maintainability and accessibility of contributor blood remain continuous difficulties that analysts and medical care suppliers keep on tending to.

In situations where hereditary elements contribute to blood problems, state-of-the-art improvements in quality treatment offer promising roads for treatment. The capacity to change or supplant broken qualities opens additional opportunities for tending to the underlying drivers of acquired blood problems. As exploration in this field advances, the potential for customized and corrective methodologies turns out to be progressively unmistakable.

Past these traditional strategies and rising advancements, for example, CRISPR-Cas9 quality altering holds groundbreaking possibilities in the domain of blood problem arrangements. The capacity to definitively alter hereditary material raises moral contemplations yet additionally opens ways to adjust hereditary irregularities at their source. The excursion toward saddling the full force of quality altering about blood problems is one of both fervor and cautious moral consultation.

Notwithstanding clinical mediations, way-of-life adjustments and steady consideration assume essential parts in overseeing blood issues. Dietary changes, actual work, and stress on the board contribute to general prosperity and can supplement clinical medicines. Schooling and support for people with blood problems and their families are fundamental parts of a complete methodology, cultivating strengthening and flexibility notwithstanding ongoing circumstances.

Cooperation between specialists, medical services suppliers, and promotion bunches is fundamental to driving advancement in the field of blood problem arrangements. By cultivating an aggregate comprehension of the difficulties presented by these circumstances, partners can cooperate to upgrade findings, further develop treatment choices, and eventually lift the personal satisfaction of people impacted by blood problems.

All in all, the scene of blood problem arrangements is developing quickly, pushed by logical forward leaps, mechanical developments, and a cooperative obligation to propel patient consideration. This presentation gives a brief look into the complex methodologies utilized to address blood problems, underscoring the continuous quest for extensive, customized, and morally sound arrangements that guarantee to reclassify the fate of hematological medication.

CHAPTER 1

Understanding Blood Disorders

Blood issues are conditions that hold portions of your blood back from going about their responsibilities. You might have a blood-coagulating jumble or a draining problem. With therapy, most blood problems become ongoing ailments that don't influence individuals' life expectancies. Treatment incorporates overseeing side effects and treating any hidden circumstances.

Blood issues are conditions that hold portions of your blood back from taking care of their responsibilities:

Your red platelets convey oxygen all through your body.

Your white platelets assist with shielding your body from disease.

Your platelets assist your blood with coagulation, so you don't drain more than typical.

Blood issues might be dangerous or noncancerous. This article centers around noncancerous blood issues.

You might acquire a noncancerous blood jumble or foster one since you have a basic condition that influences your blood.

Some blood issues may not cause side effects or require treatment. Others are constant (deep-rooted) ailments that require treatment yet regularly won't influence how long you'll live. Other blood problems are difficult ailments that can be life-threatening.

Medical care suppliers treat blood problems by overseeing side effects and treating any basic circumstances.

In all actuality, do blood problems influence my body?

By and large, noncancerous blood problems are conditions that influence your platelets and cause causes that may include:

Increment your gamble on blood clusters. Factor V Leiden, an acquired blood problem, is an illustration of a blood-thickening turmoil.
Cause you to drain more than typical in light of the fact that your blood doesn't frame blood clumps. Acquired hemophilia is an illustration of a draining problem.
What are normal blood thickening problems?
A blood-thickening confusion influences your platelets or your thickening elements (coagulation factors). Coagulation factors are proteins in your blood. Your platelets and thickening elements make blood clumps, which control dying. Blood

coagulating problems might be known as a hypercoagulable state or thrombophilia. Blood-coagulating messes include:

Prothrombin quality change: This acquired problem builds your risk of creating unusual blood clumps in your veins (profound vein apoplexy) and lungs (aspiratory embolism).

Antiphospholipid disorder: This uncommon immune system issue, which frequently influences individuals who have lupus, can cause blood clumps in a few regions of your body.

Lack of protein S: Protein S is a characteristic anticoagulant in your blood. Anticoagulants keep the blood from thickening. Protein S helps hold different proteins back from making too many blood clumps. This is an uncommonly acquired problem.

Lack of protein C: Like protein S, protein C is a characteristic anticoagulant that safeguards you from growing too many blood clusters.

Antithrombin inadequacy: This acquired problem builds your gamble of profound vein apoplexy.
Paroxysmal nighttime hemoglobinuria: This uncommon blood problem happens when your safe framework goes after your red platelets, expanding your risk of blood clumps.
Dispersed intravascular coagulation (DIC): DIC is an intriguing blood-thickening turmoil that might cause wild draining or coagulation.
Certain individuals with blood-thickening requests have an expanded risk of stroke and cardiovascular failure. Call 911 in the event that you believe you're having a pneumonic embolism since you have chest pain and trouble relaxing. Cardiovascular

failure and stroke are other ailments that need urgent treatment.

What are normal draining issues?

Draining problems happen when your blood doesn't clump ordinarily, making you drain more than expected. Draining issues include:

Von Willebrand sickness: This condition is the most widely recognized draining problem in the U.S. The vast majority of people who have von Willebrand infection acquired a transformed quality from one of their natural guardians. Certain individuals foster this condition as a result of specific tumors, immune system problems, and heart and vein illnesses.

Acquired hemophilia: This interesting hereditary condition might cause you to drain more than expected. There are three sorts of hemophilia: Type An, or exemplary hemophilia; Type B, or Christmas infection; and Type C (Rosenthal disorder).

Thrombocytopenia: This condition happens when you have a low platelet count. Invulnerable thrombocytopenia (ITP) and thrombotic thrombocytopenic purpura (TTP) are instances of illnesses that cause thrombocytopenia.

Fibrinogen inadequacy conditions: Fibrinogen is another protein that assists your blood with coagulation. On the off chance that you need more fibrinogen or your fibrinogen doesn't function as it ought to, you might have strange draining or coagulating issues.

Blood issues are conditions that hold portions of your blood back from going about their responsibilities. You might have a blood-coagulating jumble or a draining problem. With therapy, most blood problems become ongoing ailments that don't influence individuals' life expectancies. Treatment incorporates overseeing side effects and treating any hidden circumstances.

Blood issues are conditions that hold portions of your blood back from taking care of their responsibilities:

Your red platelets convey oxygen all through your body.
Your white platelets assist with shielding your body from disease.
Your platelets assist your blood with coagulation, so you don't drain more than typical.
Blood issues might be dangerous or noncancerous. This article centers around noncancerous blood issues.

You might acquire a noncancerous blood jumble or foster one since you have a basic condition that influences your blood.

Some blood issues may not cause side effects or require treatment. Others are constant (deep-rooted) ailments that require treatment yet regularly won't influence how long you'll live. Other blood problems are difficult ailments that can be life-threatening.

Medical care suppliers treat blood problems by overseeing side effects and treating any basic circumstances.

In all actuality, do blood problems influence my body?

By and large, noncancerous blood problems are conditions that influence your platelets and cause causes that may include:

Increment your gamble on blood clusters. Factor V Leiden, an acquired blood problem, is an illustration of a blood-thickening turmoil.

Cause you to drain more than typical in light of the fact that your blood doesn't frame blood clumps. Acquired hemophilia is an illustration of a draining problem.

What are normal blood thickening problems?

A blood-thickening confusion influences your platelets or your thickening elements (coagulation factors). Coagulation factors are proteins in your blood. Your platelets and thickening elements make blood clumps, which control dying. Blood coagulating problems might be known as a hypercoagulable state or thrombophilia. Blood-coagulating messes include:

Prothrombin quality change: This acquired problem builds your risk of creating unusual blood clumps in your veins (profound vein apoplexy) and lungs (aspiratory embolism).

Antiphospholipid disorder: This uncommon immune system issue, which frequently influences individuals who have lupus, can cause blood clumps in a few regions of your body.

Lack of protein S: Protein S is a characteristic anticoagulant in your blood. Anticoagulants keep blood from thickening. Protein S helps hold different proteins back from making too many blood clumps. This is an uncommonly acquired problem.

Lack of protein C: Like protein S, protein C is a characteristic anticoagulant that safeguards you from growing too many blood clusters.

Antithrombin inadequacy: This acquired problem builds your gamble of profound vein apoplexy.
Paroxysmal nighttime hemoglobinuria: This uncommon blood problem happens when your safe framework goes after your red platelets, expanding your risk of blood clumps.

Dispersed intravascular coagulation (DIC): DIC is an intriguing blood-thickening turmoil that might cause wild draining or coagulation.

Certain individuals with blood-thickening requests have an expanded risk of stroke and cardiovascular failure. Call 911 in the event that you believe you're having a pneumonic embolism since you have chest pain and trouble relaxing. Cardiovascular failure and stroke are other ailments that need crisis treatment.

What are normal draining issues?

Draining problems happen when your blood doesn't clump ordinarily, making you drain more than expected. Draining issues include:

Von Willebrand sickness: This condition is the most widely recognized draining problem in the U.S. The vast majority of people who have von Willebrand infection acquired a transformed quality from one of their natural guardians. Certain individuals foster this condition as a result of specific tumors, immune system problems, and heart and vein illnesses.

Acquired hemophilia: This interesting hereditary condition might cause you to drain more than expected. There are three sorts of hemophilia: Type An, or exemplary hemophilia; Type B, or Christmas infection; and Type C (Rosenthal disorder).

Thrombocytopenia: This condition happens when you have a low platelet count. Invulnerable thrombocytopenia (ITP) and thrombotic thrombocytopenic purpura (TTP) are instances of illnesses that cause thrombocytopenia.

Fibrinogen inadequacy conditions: Fibrinogen is another protein that assists your blood with coagulation. On the off chance that you need more fibrinogen or if your fibrinogen doesn't function as it ought to, you might have strange draining or coagulating issues.

What is the most well-known sort of blood problem?

Sickliness addresses the most well-known kind of noncancerous blood jumble. The U.S. Places for Infectious Disease Prevention and Avoidance estimates that around 3 million individuals in the U.S. have an iron deficiency of some sort. Paleness happens when you need more solid red platelets. A few sorts of paleness are acquired; however, individuals may likewise secure or foster them.

Gained anemias

Malicious paleness: Malevolent weakness, one of the reasons for a lack of vitamin B12, is an immune system condition that keeps your body from absorbing vitamin B12.

Iron-lack pallor: As its name infers, iron-inadequacy frailty happens when your body needs more iron to make hemoglobin. Red platelets need hemoglobin to convey oxygen all through your body.

Megaloblastic pallor: Megaloblastic paleness is a sort of sickness that can happen when you don't get sufficient vitamin B12 as well as nutrient B9 (folate).

Aplastic frailty: This weakness happens when undifferentiated organisms in your bone marrow don't make sufficient platelets.

Immune system hemolytic paleness: In immune system hemolytic weakness, your resistant framework goes after your red platelets.

Macrocytic paleness: This weakness happens when your bone marrow makes surprisingly enormous red platelets.

Macrocytic paleness might be brought about by myelodysplastic disorder, low folate, low B12 nutrients, liver sickness, liquor use, and certain medications.

Normocytic iron deficiency: In this sort of sickness, you have fewer red platelets than expected. There are many reasons for normocytic frailty.
Acquired anemias

Sickle cell pallor: Sickle cell iron deficiency changes your red platelets' shape, transforming round, adaptable circles into solid and tacky sickle cells that block the bloodstream.

Fanconi pallor: Fanconi iron deficiency is an uncommon blood problem. Pallor is one indication of Fanconi's iron deficiency.

Precious stone Blackfan iron deficiency: This acquired problem holds your bone marrow back from making sufficient red platelets.

Thalassemia: In thalassemia, your body delivers less hemoglobin, bringing about little red platelets and frailty.
A few sorts of iron deficiency might be acquired yet can likewise be gained:

Hemolytic frailty: In this pallor, your red platelets separate or pass on quicker than expected.
Sideroblastic weakness: Sideroblastic pallor results from unusual iron use during red platelet improvement.

Microcytic paleness: This weakness happens when your red platelets need more hemoglobin, so they're more modest than expected. Microcytic paleness happens with a lack of iron, thalassemia, sideroblastic weakness, and now and again the frailty of constant infection.

Side Effects and Causes

What are normal blood problem side effects?

Blood jumble side effects depend on the particular blood issue and its effect on your blood.

For instance, a great many people with sickliness have the accompanying side effects:

Exhaustion and shortcomings.
Tipsiness.
Skin that is paler than expected.
Quick heartbeat (heart palpitations).
Windedness.
Normal draining issues have side effects
The most widely recognized side effect is extreme and persistent death. You might need to converse with your medical care supplier, assuming you have any of the accompanying side effects:

Nosebleeds: These are nosebleeds that last longer than 10 minutes and happen at least five times each year.

Extreme dying: Cuts or wounds that drain longer than 10 minutes.

Interior dying: This might cause joint torment.

Wounds: Swelling that occurs for reasons unknown or after a minor injury.

Post-medical procedure dying: Weighty draining after any sort of medical procedure, including dental medical procedures.
Weighty periods (feminine dying): This is draining that is so heavy that you really want to change your cushion or tampon consistently or have draining that endures longer than seven days.

Weighty draining after labor or premature delivery.

Blood in crap (stool): Blood in your crap or draining in the wake of crapping might be a side effect of other ailments. Converse with your medical services supplier on the off chance that you have blood in your crap.
Blood in pee (hematuria): Converse with your medical care supplier assuming you notice blood when you pee, especially in the event that you have a critical need to pee and there's blood in your pee.
Normal blood coagulating jumble side effects
Blood-coagulating messes increase your risk of creating blood clumps in your veins, lungs, and different regions of your body. Individuals with blood thickening problems might have the accompanying side effects:

Expanding, delicacy, and agony in your leg can mean you have profound vein apoplexy.

Chest torment with windedness can mean a potential pneumonic embolism.
Coronary failure.
Stroke.

Findings and Tests
How do medical care suppliers analyze blood problems?
Medical care suppliers will do actual assessments and get some information about your clinical history and your side effects. They might do a few blood tests.

Red platelet tests
Red platelets convey oxygen from your lungs to your body's tissues. Your tissues produce energy with the oxygen and deliver carbon dioxide. Your red platelets take the carbon dioxide waste to your lungs for you to breathe out.

Suppliers will take blood tests to assess your red platelet count and your red platelet parts. They might do tests to see what your red platelets resemble under a magnifying instrument. Red platelet tests might include:

Hemoglobin test: Hemoglobin is the principal part of red platelets. The test is frequently used to recognize pallor.

Hematocrit test: This test estimates the level of red platelets in your blood.

Reticulocyte count: Reticulocytes are juvenile red platelets. This test verifies whether your bone marrow is delivering sufficient sound red platelets.
White platelet tests
White platelets address around 1% of your blood. They safeguard your body against contamination. Unusual white platelet levels might be indications of a few ailments.

For instance, a high white platelet count (leukocytosis) may mean you have contamination, irritation, or malignant

growth. A low white platelet count (leukopenia) might be an indication of conditions ranging from a lack of nutrients to disease. Hemolytic frailty: In this pallor, your red platelets separate or pass on quicker than expected.
Sideroblastic weakness: Sideroblastic pallor results from unusual iron use during red platelet improvement.

Microcytic paleness: This weakness happens when your red platelets need more hemoglobin, so they're more modest than expected. Microcytic paleness happens with lack of iron, thalassemia, sideroblastic weakness, and now and again frailty of constant infection.

Side Effects and Causes

What are normal blood problem side effects?

Blood jumble side effects depend on the particular blood issue and its effect on your blood.

For instance, a great many people with sickliness have the accompanying side effects:

Exhaustion and shortcomings.
Tipsiness.
Skin that is paler than expected.
Quick heartbeat (heart palpitations).
Windedness.
Normal draining issues have side effects
The most widely recognized side effect is extreme and persistent death. You might need to converse with your medical care supplier, assuming you have any of the accompanying side effects:

Nosebleeds: These are nosebleeds that last longer than 10 minutes and happen at least five times each year.

Extreme dying: cuts or wounds that drain longer than 10 minutes.

Interior dying: This might cause joint torment.

Wounds: Swelling that occurs for reasons unknown or after a minor injury.

Post-medical procedure dying: Weighty draining after any sort of medical procedure, including dental medical procedures.
Weighty periods (feminine dying): This is draining that is so heavy that you really want to change your cushion or tampon consistently or have draining that endures longer than seven days.
Weighty draining after labor or premature delivery.

Blood in crap (stool): Blood in your crap or draining in the wake of crapping might be a side effect of other ailments. Converse with your medical services supplier on the off chance that you have blood in your crap.

Blood in pee (hematuria): Converse with your medical care supplier assuming you notice blood when you pee, especially in the event that you have a critical need to pee and there's blood in your pee.

Normal blood coagulating jumble side effects

Blood-coagulating messes increase your risk of creating blood clumps in your veins, lungs, and different regions of your body. Individuals with blood thickening problems might have the accompanying side effects:

Expanding, delicacy, and agony in your leg can mean you have profound vein apoplexy.

Chest torment with windedness can mean a potential pneumonic embolism.

Coronary failure.

Stroke.

Findings and Tests

How do medical care suppliers analyze blood problems?
Medical care suppliers will do actual assessments and get some information about your clinical history and your side effects. They might do a few blood tests.

Red platelet tests
Red platelets convey oxygen from your lungs to your body's tissues. Your tissues produce energy with the oxygen and deliver carbon dioxide. Your red platelets take the carbon dioxide waste to your lungs for you to breathe out.

Suppliers will take blood tests to assess your red platelet count and your red platelet parts. They might do tests to see what your red platelets resemble under a magnifying instrument. Red platelet tests might include:

Hemoglobin test: Hemoglobin is the principal part of red platelets. The test is frequently used to recognize pallor.

Hematocrit test: This test estimates the level of red platelets in your blood.

Reticulocyte count: Reticulocytes are juvenile red platelets. This test verifies whether your bone marrow is delivering sufficient sound red platelets.
White platelet tests
White platelets address around 1% of your blood. They safeguard your body against contamination. Unusual white platelet levels might be indications of a few ailments.

For instance, a high white platelet count (leukocytosis) may mean you have contamination, irritation, or malignant growth. A low white platelet count (leukopenia) might be an indication of conditions ranging from a lack of nutrients to disease.

There are three sorts of white platelets — granulocytes, monocytes, and lymphocytes. Granulocytes incorporate three sub-sorts of white platelets — eosinophils, basophils, and neutrophils. Your medical care supplier might do a total blood count (CBC) with differential to assess each white platelet type:

Eosinophils: Eosinophils shield your body from diseases. Blood tests might show high eosinophil levels (eosinophilia). Eosinophilia might be an indication of hidden ailments.
Basophils: Basophils safeguard your body against allergens and different gatecrashers. Basophilia happens when your body delivers such a large number of basophils. A high basophil count might be an indication of specific blood diseases.

Neutrophils: Neutrophils are the most widely recognized white platelet type. Neutrophils are the people on call for battle contamination. Low neutrophil counts are neutropenia. Neutropenia might increase your risk of serious disease.

Monocytes: These white platelets find and annihilate microorganisms. Elevated levels of monocytes (monocytosis) might be an indication of irresistible infections.

Lymphocytes: There are two fundamental sorts of lymphocytes: T lymphocytes (White blood cells) deal with your body's resistant framework reaction. They assault and obliterate tainted cells and different interlopers; B lymphocytes (B cells) make antibodies. Antibodies are proteins that target infections, microscopic organisms, and other unfamiliar trespassers.
Platelet tests
Platelets, additionally called thrombocytes, assist with making blood clusters and

controlling dying. Tests to assess your platelet well-being might include:

Platelet count: This test estimates the quantity of platelets in your blood.
Mean platelet volume (MPV) test: This blood test estimates the typical size of your platelets.
Fringe blood smear (PBS): Your supplier might utilize this test to look at your platelets under a magnifying lens. (They likewise utilize this test to inspect your white and red platelets.)

The executives and Treatment
How do medical service suppliers treat blood issues?
By and large, medical service suppliers center around recognizing and treating hidden conditions that cause blood problems. They likewise treat blood jumble side effects. Medicines might include:

Vigilant pausing: Some blood problems don't cause observable side effects. Assuming that that is what is happening, your supplier will screen your general well-being, giving close consideration to any new signs or side effects that you're fostering a blood problem.

Blood and platelet bondings: Suppliers might utilize blood bondings to help reduce platelet levels for individuals with serious types of iron deficiency. They might utilize platelet bonding to assist with blood thickening issues.

Anticoagulants: These medications assist with blood thickening issues by holding your blood back from coagulating too, without any problems.

Development factor supplementation: This treatment invigorates your bone marrow, so it makes extra red and white platelets. Erythropoietin-invigorating specialists (ESA) are instances of development factor supplements.

Corticosteroids: This treatment smothers your safe framework. Suppliers might use steroids to treat immune system hemolytic weakness.

These medicines have different side effects. Get some information about the treatment's incidental effects. They'll assist you with overseeing them.

Counteraction

Will individuals forestall noncancerous blood problems?

That depends on the particular issue. Some blood problems are acquired, and that implies you can't forestall them. Others are brought about by basic circumstances that you might possibly have the option to forestall. While you can't necessarily forestall blood problems, there are steps you can take to diminish your risk of creating confusion.

How might I lessen my risk of fostering these problems?

Dealing with your general well-being might decrease your risk of creating conditions that cause blood problems. Ideas include:

Eat a sound eating routine abundant in nutrients and minerals: This incorporates food sources with iron, for example, eggs, turkey, lean hamburgers, and organ meats like kidney and liver. Vegetables, including dark beans, verdant green vegetables, and earthy-colored rice, are different food varieties that assist with expanding your iron intake.

Remain dynamic: Normal activity helps support your resistant framework.

Keep a sound weight: Converse with a medical services supplier about achieving and keeping a weight that is ideal for you.

Do whatever it takes to forestall contamination: Make certain to clean up well and frequently. Consult with your supplier about the occasional influenza shot (antibody) and some other immunizations you ought to consider.

Get normal exams: In the event that you have a blood issue or you might be in danger of fostering a blood problem, your supplier will make customary arrangements to really take a look at your general well-being. They might do blood tests.

Standpoint/Visualization

What is the anticipated or expected result for noncancerous blood problems?

Non-dangerous blood issues differ broadly. For instance, many individuals with blood-thickening problems might have ordinary life expectancies but may require drugs and treatment until the end of their lives. However, some blood problems, similar to sickle cell iron deficiency, might be life-threatening. Individuals' guesses additionally rely upon variables like their age and, generally speaking, their well-being. On the off chance that you have a blood issue, ask your medical services supplier what you can anticipate.

How would you live with a blood problem? Blood problems might significantly have an impact on your lifestyle. In any case, there are things you can do to keep up with your personal satisfaction. For instance:

Teach your loved ones: Make sense of what your blood issue might mean for you. Like that, they'll comprehend the reason why you will be unable to do specific exercises, and they'll have at least some idea of what to do in the event that you have a health-related crisis.

Think about wearing a clinical-ready wristband: In cases of extreme ailment or injury, wearing this wristband educates medical service suppliers concerning your condition so they can give you the consideration you want.

Eat an iron-rich eating routine: Eating a solid eating routine can help anybody living with a blood problem.

Treat any draining immediately: In the event that you have a draining problem, your medical services supplier might recommend a drug (factor) to assist your blood with coagulation. Individuals with draining problems ought to treat draining rapidly by accepting drugs as recommended. Diminish your risk of injury: On the off chance that you have a draining issue, stay away from physical games that might increase your risk of falling or being hit. Continuously wear your safety belt. On the off chance that you ride a bicycle, wear a head protector.

Contact your medical services supplier if you notice changes in your body that might be signs your condition is deteriorating.

When would it be advisable for me to go to the trauma center?
Some noncancerous blood problems might cause health-related crises. Individuals with blood-coagulating diseases have an

expanded risk of blood clusters that might cause pneumonic embolism, cardiovascular failure, and stroke. In the event that you have blood-thickening confusion and have chest torment, call 911.

On the off chance that you have a draining issue and you're harmed, you might experience difficulty controlling your dying. In the event that your endorsed medicine doesn't slow your bloodstream, go to the trauma center.

What inquiries would it be a good idea for me to pose to my medical care supplier?
There are numerous sorts of noncancerous blood issues. Assuming that you've been determined to have one of these issues, you might need to pose your supplier with the accompanying inquiries:

What sort of blood problem do I have?
What will this condition mean for me?
Is this condition perilous?

What are medicines?

What are the treatment's aftereffects?

Will treatment fix me?

In the event that not, will I generally need to take drugs?
How could I foster this blood problem?
Assuming that I acquired this turmoil, should my nearby relatives undergo hereditary testing?

Non-carcinogenic blood issues are conditions that keep your blood from going about its business. Your blood may not make blood clumps to hold you back from draining more than ordinary. Your blood might make clusters too effectively, expanding your risk of blood clumps that could cause a stroke or respiratory failure.

Frequently, these circumstances are persistent (long-haul) and require deep-rooted clinical consideration. With therapy, the vast majority of people with noncancerous blood issues have an ordinary life expectancy and great personal satisfaction.

CHAPTER 2

Types And Classification Of Blood Disorders

Individuals might be impacted by various sorts of blood conditions and diseases. Normal blood issues incorporate pallor and draining problems, for example, hemophilia, blood clumps, and blood diseases like leukemia, lymphoma, and myeloma.

When something is the matter with your blood, it can influence your absolute well-being. To that end, you should be aware of a portion of the normal blood issues that might influence you.

Conversing with your primary care physician is the initial step to take if you accept you might have a blood condition. On the off chance that you are determined to have a blood issue, your primary care physician might refer you to a hematologist.

Hematology is the investigation of blood for well-being and illness. It incorporates issues with the red platelets, white platelets, platelets, veins, bone marrow, lymph hubs, spleen, and the proteins associated with draining and coagulating (hemostasis and apoplexy). A hematologist is a clinical expert who applies this specific data to treat patients with blood conditions.

Characterizations for hematological neoplasms depend on World Wellbeing Association distributions (13, 14), which frame the global principles for appraisal and determination of hematological neoplasms. Utilization of the WHO standards relies upon the clinical history and actual assessment, morphology (cytology or histology), immunophenotyping, cytogenetic examination, and, in certain conditions, atomic hereditary examination. The past French-American-English (FAB) bunch orders might be utilized (1) when these methods are not all free and (2) in making a temporary morphological finding (for example, in intense leukemia) while anticipating the consequences of additional tests. Whichever grouping is utilized, the standards ought to be completely noticed with the goal that there is consistency between various focuses and nations. The WHO grouping of hematological neoplasms has a few significant classifications.

The WHO grouping arranges cases as AML if the accompanying rules are met:

1.
There are something like 20% of shoot cells of myeloid genealogy in the blood, bone marrow or

2.

On the off chance that the erythroid cells are no less than half of bone marrow cells, impact cells are somewhere around 20% of nonerythroid cells or

3.

Crude erythroid cells comprise no less than 80% of bone marrow cells or

4.

One of various determined chromosomal adjustments is available.

It ought to be noticed that the WHO order is varyingly leveled. If suitable, cases are first allocated to the classification of treatment-related leukemia. Then, cases are appointed, if proper, to the classification of AML with intermittent hereditary anomalies. Cases keep on being appointed to progressive classes, with residual cases at long last being arranged as 'AML, not in any case determined.' Blastic plasmacytoid dendritic cell neoplasms and myeloid neoplasms related to Down syndrome are perceived as unambiguous elements.

WHO order of the myelodysplastic conditions (MDS)

2008 WHO classification Terminology proposed for the 2016 update of the WHO order
Hard-headed cytopenia with unilineage dysplasia
Hard-headed frailty
Hard-headed neutropenia
Hard-headed thrombocytopenia MDS and single ancestry dysplasia
Hard-headed frailty with ring sideroblasts MDS with single ancestry dysplasia and ring sideroblasts
Recalcitrant cytopenia with multilineage dysplasia (regardless of ring sideroblasts) MDS with multilineage dysplasia

MDS with multilineage dysplasia and ring sideroblasts

Recalcitrant pallor with overabundance impacts 1 MDS with abundance impacts 1

Recalcitrant pallor with overabundance impacts 2 MDS with abundance impacts 2

Myelodysplastic condition with secluded del (5q) Myelodysplastic disorder with detached del (5q)

Myelodysplastic condition, unclassifiable Myelodysplastic disorder, unclassifiable

Adolescence has a myelodysplastic condition

Temporary element: stubborn cytopenia of childhood Childhood myelodysplastic condition

Temporary element: stubborn cytopenia of experience growing up

The WHO grouping of intense leukemia (15) records cytogenetic irregularities that, in the mix with $\geq$ 20 impacts, demonstrate a conclusion of AML with myelodysplasia-related change.

The WHO grouping expects that intense leukemia should be demonstrated to be lymphoid before it is ordered as ALL. This characterization gathers ALL and lymphoblastic lymphoma, utilizing the assignments B lymphoblastic leukemia/lymphoma and T lymphoblastic leukemia/lymphoma. These assignments are too unwieldy to even consider involving in clinical practice and without a doubt, hematologists will keep on alluding to 'intense lymphoblastic leukemia.' The FAB characterization of Everything is currently repetitive, except that FAB L3 morphology (for example, the presence of'shoot cells' with basophilic cytoplasm and vacuolation) is of extensive clinical importance and ought to be perceived. In the vast majority of these cases, the phones are immunologically full-grown, communicating surface layer immunoglobulin, and the condition addresses a leukemic form of Burkill lymphoma. The WHO categorization of such cases as lymphoma is more proper than being sorted as ALL and is clinically significant because the treatment is earnest and varies impressively from the treatment of ALL.

CHAPTER 3

Causes And Risk Factors

A larger part of blood problems are brought about by transformations in pieces of explicit qualities that can be passed down in families. A few ailments, drugs, and way of life variables can likewise create blood issues.

Blood infections and problems influence at least one piece of the blood and keep your blood from taking care of its business. Many blood illnesses and problems are brought about by qualities. Different causes incorporate different illnesses, results of medications, and an absence of specific supplements in your eating regimen.

Normal blood issues incorporate paleness and draining problems like hemophilia.

Inherited draining problems happen because of the nonappearance or lack of explicit coagulation proteins. The three most normal genetic draining problems are hemophilia A (factor VIII lack), hemophilia B (factor IX inadequacy), and von Willebrand sickness.

Platelet problems are the most widely recognized reason for draining issues and are generally procured as opposed to acquired.

Am I In danger?

Draining issues like hemophilia and von Willebrand's sickness result when the blood misses the mark on thickening elements. These illnesses are quite often acquired, albeit in uncommon cases they can be fostered sometime down the road assuming the body structures antibodies that battle against the blood's regular thickening variables. People and pregnant ladies with a family background of draining problems ought to converse with their primary care physicians about recognition and treatment. Side effects of draining issues might include:

Simple swelling
Draining gums
Weighty draining from little cuts or dental work
Unexplained nosebleeds
Weighty feminine dying
Seeping into joints
Over-the-top draining following a medical procedure

Hemophilia is an uncommon, acquired draining problem that can go from gentle to extreme, contingent upon how much coagulation factor is available in the blood. Hemophilia is named type A or type B, in light of which kind of coagulation factor is deficient with regards to (factor VIII in type An and consider IX sort B). Hemophilia results from a hereditary deformity tracked down on the X chromosome. Ladies have two X chromosomes. Ladies who have one X chromosome with imperfect quality are named transporters and they can pass the sickness onto their children. Because of irregular chromosome enactment, a few ladies transporters might go from asymptomatic to suggestive relying upon the amount of their variable VIII or IX is inactivated. A few ladies might have "gentle hemophilia," however this is more uncommon. Men have one X and one Y chromosome, so assuming their X chromosome has the blemished quality, they will have hemophilia.

Since blood doesn't cluster as expected without sufficient coagulation factor, any cut or injury conveys the gamble of unnecessary dying. Furthermore, individuals with hemophilia might experience the ill effects of inner draining that can harm joints, organs, and tissues over the long run.

Previously, individuals with hemophilia were treated with bondings of component VIII acquired from donor blood, yet by the mid-1980s, these items were found to communicate blood-borne infections, including hepatitis and HIV. Because of further developed screening procedures and a significant advancement that empowered researchers to make manufactured blood factors in the lab by cloning the qualities liable for explicit thickening elements, the present component substitution treatments are unadulterated and a lot more secure than any time in recent memory.

Normal blood issues incorporate pallor, draining problems, for example, hemophilia, blood clusters, and blood tumors like leukemia, lymphoma, and myeloma.

AILMENTS THAT CAN CAUSE A LOW PLATELET COUNT

A low platelet count might happen due to trusted Sources:

the bone marrow not creating an adequate number of platelets
the body annihilating or spending the platelets that the bone marrow produces
the spleen clutching such a large number of platelets, implying that the sum in the blood is excessively low
Certain ailments can likewise cause an individual to have a low platelet count. These include:

Aplastic iron deficiency: This intriguing blood condition happens when the bone marrow stops making satisfactory fresh blood cells.

Immune system illnesses: Certain immune system infections can erroneously assault an individual's safe framework and obliterate their platelets. Infections that can do this incorporate idiopathic thrombocytopenic purpura (ITP), lupus, and rheumatoid joint pain.

Cancer: A few malignant growths, like leukemia or lymphoma, can harm bone marrow and obliterate blood foundational microorganisms. This can make the undifferentiated organisms stop developing sound platelets. Some disease therapies, including radiation treatment and chemotherapy, may likewise annihilate foundational microorganisms.

Conditions that cause blood clumps: A few circumstances cause blood clusters to form. These circumstances incorporate thrombotic thrombocytopenic purpura (TTP) and scattered intravascular coagulation (DIC). These circumstances can make the body utilize accessible platelets in general, prompting a low platelet count.

Infections: Bacterial or viral contaminants may briefly bring down a platelet count.

Huge spleen: On the off chance that an individual's spleen is huge, it might store a large number of platelets. This can cause a low platelet count in the blood.

Surgery: At times, counterfeit heart valves, vein units, or machines and tubing for blood bondings or sidestepping a medical procedure might obliterate platelets.

Pregnancy can at times make an individual foster gentle thrombocytopenia. The specific justification for this is obscure; however, it is, by all accounts, more normal near conveyance.

CHAPTER 4

Diagnostic Approaches In Identifying Blood Disorders

Your primary care physician might arrange a few tests, including a total blood count (CBC), to determine the number of each kind of platelet you have. Your primary care physician may likewise arrange a bone marrow biopsy to check whether there are any strange cells in your marrow. This will include eliminating a modest quantity of bone marrow for testing.

A strange blood count or platelet morphology doesn't guarantee to demonstrate an essential hematology issue since it might mirror a hidden non hematological condition or might be the consequence of remedial medications.

Paleness happens in many circumstances, yet an essential blood sickness ought to be looked at when a patient has splenomegaly, lymphadenopathy, a draining propensity or apoplexy, or potentially vague side effects (disquietude, sweats, or weight reduction).

Likewise with any clinical issue, the most vital phases in deciding the determination incorporate getting a cautious clinical and drug history and an exhaustive actual assessment. The consequences of these, mixed with the patient's age, sex, ethnic beginning, social and family ancestry, and information on the locally prominent illnesses, will determine the ensuing research facility examinations.

Although the scope of hematological tests accessible to help clinical and general well-being administrations is expansive, frequently the least difficult examinations are most valuable in showing the conclusion. Indeed, even inadequately resourced research centers are generally ready to give an underlying set of tests like hemoglobin focus (Hb), white platelet count (WBC), and platelet count

An examination of a thought-draining issue requires a down-to-earth technique that believes the clinical issue to be researched, the pretest likelihood of genuine positive and bogus positive discoveries, the examinations can be performed locally or in a reference lab, and breaking point the number of blood tests expected to lay out a finding. It is frequently worthwhile to test for von Willebrand sickness and platelet capability problems and for coagulation absconds, including fibrinogen issues. An examination for more extraordinary draining problems, including those influencing factor XIII, α2 antiplasmin, and plasminogen activator inhibitor-1, is suitable when confronted with an extreme innate or acquired draining issue that can't be made sense of by the underlying symptomatic examinations.

We carried out a normalized approach for assessing draining problems quite a long time ago that worked with an assessment of the responsiveness and particularity of individual tests and test boards for draining issues.

counting follow-up tests to think about after beginning examinations. Both inherent and gained draining confusion can be drawn closer by this methodology.

While smoothed-out testing is frequently useful, there are circumstances that require an individualized methodology. A genuine model is the symptomatic testing of a rope blood test for a particular problem that influences the infant's parent or sibling(sng(s). Another model is focusing on examinations when a youngster is excessively little to draw the volume of blood required for complete examinations. More uncommon, autosomal passive draining problems merit more prominent thought when the patient is from a locale with a high pervasiveness of interesting problems or a culture that acknowledges relationships. Gained VW condition (AVWS) and procured platelet capability problems are often thought of in patients with a hidden blood issue (e.g., a myeloproliferative or lymphoproliferative neoplasm, monoclonal gammopathy) or different circumstances (e.g., stenosis of the aortic valve). The elderly are at a higher risk for autoantibody-instigated diseases, including procured hemophilia, factor V inadequacy, XIII lack, and AVWS from a monoclonal gammopathy.

For most patients that require a draining problem assessment, we all the while test for (I) coagulation deformities and fibrinogen issues, utilizing the prothrombin time (PT)/globally standardized proportion

(INR), enacted fractional thromboplastin time (APTT), thrombin time, and Clauss fibrinogen measure; and (ii) VWD and platelet capability issues (Figure 1), utilizing VWD screens, light transmission platelet aggregometry (LTA), and frequently, entire mount electron microscopy (EM) to survey for platelet thick granule lack. This system distinguishes the more normal draining problems that debilitate essential hemostasis or potentially cause coagulation test irregularities

in all kinds of people. It thinks that autosomal predominant draining problems (e.g., many types of VWD and platelet capability issues, dysfibrinogenemia) and X-connected messes (i.e., hemophilia) are more normal than autosomal latent draining issues. We utilize auxiliary examinations to affirm and additionally research irregularities identified by the underlying examinations, assuming the discoveries were negative, to assess for draining issues that were not evaluated. This methodology is extensively relevant, in spite of the fact that it might require customization, in view of which tests are privately endorsed and approved and should be possible somewhere else.

We have found it valuable to examine with the patient the number of test draws and visits that are ordinarily expected to finish tests for draining problems (generally 2-3). We likewise talk about how no reason might be found, in light of the fact that mucocutaneous draining issues of unsure reason are very normal. Assuming an individual with critical draining issues has made nondiagnostic discoveries, we consider the conclusions that might have been neglected and ought to be barred.

Coagulation evaluating tests for the underlying workup of a draining issue

It is a far-reaching practice to incorporate a PT/INR and an APTT in draining problem examination to assess for possible irregularities and lay out a pattern in the event that the individual drains and fosters a dilutional coagulopathy.

A thrombin time and a Clauss (cuttable) fibrinogen assurance ought to be remembered for starting examinations to guarantee that fibrinogen issues are sufficiently recognized, On the off chance that the discoveries recommend a fibrinogen problem, we assess fibrinogen antigen levels and play out a Reptilase time to help recognize hypo-, dys-, and afibrinogenemia. 13 As dysfibrinogenemia is autosomal dominant, family concentrates frequently reveal extra cases, in some cases with negligible draining side effects.

At the point when the thrombin time is delayed and the PT/INR, APTT, and fibrinogen are ordinary, it is critical to consider drug-initiated surrenders. Strangely, valproic corrosive treatment is one of the more normal reasons for a detached, delayed thrombin time among people trying to treat draining disorders. 1. Medication impacts need to be thought about while draining problem examinations are mentioned after anticoagulation treatment is begun (e.g., to keep a stroke from atrial fibrillation) to additionally evaluate gambles/benefits as a result of earlier draining side effects that had not been researched (e.g., menorrhagia, unusual swelling, or over the top draining with careful/dental and different difficulties). In the event that a doctor orders draining confusion examinations on a patient taking an immediate thrombin or variable Xa inhibitor, they ought to request that the patient take their morning portion of anticoagulation after the examinations are attended to restrict drug obstruction.

CHAPTER 5

Treatments And Therapies

At Fred Hutchinson Malignant Growth Community, our elite specialists give thorough, group-based therapy for blood diseases and different issues that influence the blood, bone marrow, or resistant framework.

Being determined to have a blood problem can feel overpowering. We have an accomplished, merciful group prepared to help.

Fred Cubby has hematologists and hematologist-oncologists who work in blood malignant growths and nonmalignant blood illnesses; the most progressive demonstrative, treatment, and recuperation programs; and broad help.

Inventive Blood Issue Treatments

Our patient's approach progressed treatments, incorporating those being investigated in clinical examinations directed here and at UW Medication. Our doctors and researchers have spearheaded many blood problems medicines, and we advance new treatments consistently.

Blood Confusion Treatment Custom-made to You

Your Fred Pen group fosters an individualized treatment plan for you in view of your particular illness, its seriousness, how it has advanced, your age, your general well-being, and your family ancestry. We join these variables with the most recent logical information and our experience treating numerous others who've confronted a similar disease.

Alongside your hematologist or hematologist-oncologist, medical attendants, and medical attendant caseworkers, we'll include extra specialists who spend significant time treating individuals with blood problems and disease in the event that you want them—specialists like a radiation oncologist, social laborer, actual specialist, palliative consideration expert, or dietitian.

During and after therapy, your group gives follow-up care as well as help on a timetable custom-made for you. We comprehend that your sickness and therapy could affect essentially every part of your life, and we're here to assist you with adapting to the physical, useful, and profound impacts.

The doctors at Fred Box treat an extensive variety of blood issues, utilizing the most recent treatments, with the end goal of giving consideration to your overall individual. We'll obviously make sense of every one of your choices, including which treatment course we accept is best for you and why.

Contingent upon your specific analysis, treatment could include:

Development elements to invigorate platelet creation
Steroids or different medications to smother your insusceptible framework
Chemotherapy to obliterate strange cells
Bonding to help you with sound platelets
Quality treatment to supplant or deactivate an illness causing quality or to present an infection battling quality
Immunotherapy is the force of your own invulnerable framework to battle infection.

Treatment for Blood Issues

At Fred Hutchinson Malignant Growth Place, our top-notch specialists give thorough, group-based therapy for blood tumors and different problems that influence the blood, bone marrow, or safe framework.

Being determined to have a blood problem can feel overpowering. We have an accomplished, merciful group prepared to help.

ON THIS PAGE
Fred Pen Blood Problems Skill | Treatment Choices

Blood Problems Skill at Fred Cubby
All that You Really Want is Here
Fred Pen has hematologists and hematologist-oncologists who work in blood malignant growths and nonmalignant blood illnesses; the most progressive

demonstrative, therapy, and recuperation programs; and broad help.

Inventive Blood Issue Treatments

Our patient's approach progressed treatments, incorporating those being investigated in clinical examinations directed here and at UW Medication. Our doctors and researchers have spearheaded many blood problems medicines, and we advance new treatments consistently.

Blood Turmoil Treatment Customized to You

Your Fred Box group fosters an individualized treatment plan for you in light of your particular sickness, its seriousness, how it has advanced, your age, your general well-being, and your family ancestry. We consolidate these variables with the most recent logical information and our experience treating numerous others who've confronted a similar disease.

Group Based Approach

Alongside your hematologist or hematologist-oncologist, medical caretakers, and medical attendant caseworker, we'll include extra specialists who have some expertise in treating individuals with blood problems and malignant growth in the event that you want them—specialists like a radiation oncologist, social laborer, actual specialist, palliative consideration expert, or dietitian.

Progressing Care and Backing
During and after therapy, your group gives follow-up care as well as help on a timetable customized to you. We comprehend that your infection and treatment could influence virtually every part of your life, and we're here to assist you with adapting to the physical, reasonable, and close-to-home impacts.
Treatment Choices

The doctors at Fred Pen treat an extensive variety of blood issues, utilizing the most recent treatments, with the end goal of giving consideration to you in general. We'll obviously make sense of every one of your choices, including which treatment course we accept is best for you and why.

Contingent upon your specific analysis, treatment could include:

Development elements to invigorate platelet creation
Steroids or different medications to smother your insusceptible framework
Chemotherapy to obliterate strange cells
Bonding to help you with solid platelets
Quality treatment to supplant or deactivate an illness causing quality or to present an infection battling quality
Immunotherapy to saddle the force of your own safe framework to battle infection

Study Immunotherapy

Draining problems like hemophilia might call for blood-part treatments like platelet bonding or coagulating factors. Sicknesses that include coagulating could require drugs that decrease the risk of clump framing.

A few circumstances require a bone marrow relocation to supply your marrow undifferentiated organisms with solid ones. Doctors at the Fred Pen Blood and Marrow Relocate Program have performed in excess of 17,500 bone marrow transfers—more than any other establishment on the planet.

Blood bonding is a typical, safe operation wherein blood is given to you through an intravenous, or IV, line embedded in one of your veins. This treatment additionally gives blood on the off chance that your body isn't making blood as expected all alone.

Four sorts of blood items might be given through blood bonding:

Entire blood

Red platelets are the platelets that convey oxygen all through the body

Platelets are platelet pieces that assist your blood with thickening

Plasma, the liquid piece of blood

The greater part of the blood utilized for bonding comes from entire blood gifts given by volunteer blood benefactors. At times, individuals have their own blood gathered and put away half a month prior to an elective medical procedure on the off chance that it is required.

After a specialist discovers that you want a blood bond, your blood will be tested to ensure that the blood you are given is a decent match. Blood bondings, for the most part, require 1 to 4 hours to finish. You will be observed during and after the technique.

Blood bondings are generally extremely safe in light of the fact that giving blood is painstakingly tried, taken care of, and put away. Nonetheless, there is a little opportunity that your body might have a gentle or even an extreme response to the benefactor's blood.

Different difficulties with blood bonding might include:

Fever
Heart or lung issues
Alloimmunization, when the body's regular protection framework assaults platelets
Interesting yet serious responses were given when white platelets assaulted your body's solid tissues
Certain individuals likewise have medical conditions from getting an excessive amount of iron after continuous bonding. There is likewise a tiny possibility of getting an irresistible illness like hepatitis B or C or HIV through blood bonding. For HIV, that opportunity is under 1 of every 1 million. Logical examination and cautious clinical

controls make the inventory of given blood extremely protected.

Blood or bone marrow transfers are performed in an emergency clinic. Frequently, you should remain in the medical clinic for one to about fourteen days before the transfer to get ready. You will get exceptional medications and perhaps radiation to annihilate your unusually immature microorganisms and debilitate your insusceptible framework before the transfer, with the goal that your body won't dismiss the contributor cells after the transfer.

Upon the arrival of the transfer, you will be conscious and might be given medication to loosen up during the process. The undeveloped cells will be given to you through an IV (intravenous catheter). The immature microorganisms venture out through your blood to your bone marrow, where they start making new solid platelets.

At the point when the solid foundational microorganisms come from you, the methodology is called an autologous transfer. At the point when the undeveloped cells come from someone else, called a contributor, it is an allogeneic transfer. For allogeneic transfers, specialists attempt to find a donor whose platelets are the best counterpart for you. Your primary care physician will think about utilizing cells from your nearby relatives, from individuals who are not connected with you and who have enlisted with the Public Marrow Contributor Program, or from openly putting away umbilical line blood.

Your medical care supplier will continue to watch your recuperation, as a rule, for as long as one year or more. After the transfer, your blood counts will be checked habitually to see whether fresh blood cells have begun to fill in your bone marrow. The length of your recovery depends on many variables.

Before you leave the clinic, you will get itemized directions on the most proficient method to forestall disease and different entanglements.

Despite the fact that blood or bone marrow relocation is a powerful treatment for certain circumstances, the method can cause inconveniences.

The expected medications and radiation before your transfer can cause incieffects,effects including:

Queasiness
Spewing
Loose bowels
Sluggishness
Mouth sore
Skin rashes
Balding
Liver harm
These therapies can debilitate your body's regular guards against microbes and

disorders and raise your risk of contamination.

After relocating, certain individuals might encounter a serious inconvenience called unite versus sickness, which is the point at which the given undeveloped cells assault the body. In different cases, the body might dismiss the contributor of immature microorganisms after the transfer, which can be a very difficult process.

The accompanying medications might assist with treating your draining issue.

Antifibrinolytic specialists, for example, tranexamic corrosives, assist with treating draining after labor or during dental work and different techniques.
Conception prevention pills can assist with bringing down weighty feminine draining in VWD.

Desmopressin (DDAVP), a human-made chemical, can assist with halting minor draining in hemophilia or VWD.

Immunosuppressive medications, for example, prednisone, assist with obstructing the creation of antibodies, causing draining issues. Incidental effects can include contamination and diabetes.
Monoclonal antibodies can emulate the missing variable to assist with blood structure clusters. For instance, emicizumab is an immune response that scaffolds factors IX and X to impersonate the manner in which factor VIII works, which can assist with treating individuals with hemophilia A.
Vitamin K enhancements treat the lack of vitamin K.

Factor substitution treatment

Factor substitution treatment is a kind of treatment where thickening variables that are from blood gifts or made in a lab are given to supplant the missing coagulation factor. Your medical services supplier might suggest factor substitution treatment when you experience draining or to keep draining from happening. Treatment with substitution treatment consistently to forestall draining is called prophylactic treatment.

Factor substitution treatment might incorporate various parts.

Thickening variable concentrates supplant the missing coagulation factor in your blood. This treatment can raise the risk of creating antibodies that block coagulation factors, which can make your draining problem harder to treat. Now and then, consider concentrating higher sums, which can in any case assist with treating draining issues connected with antibodies.
New frozen plasma, from human blood, contains all the thickening elements. It can assist with treating the draining issues that happen while numerous coagulation factors

are missing, for example, liver illness-related dying.

By passing, specialists can assist your blood with coagulation when antibodies that block thickening variables are causing your draining issue. This treatment can raise the risk of blood clusters framing in the veins.

CHAPTER 6

Nutritional Strategies to Support Blood Health

Following these nourishing methodologies can help you diminish or try to kill some gambling factors, like lessening aggregate and LDL-cholesterol; bringing down pulse, blood sugars, and fatty oils and decreasing body weight. While most dietary plans let you know what you can't eat (as a rule your number one food source!), the most remarkable sustenance methodologies assist you with zeroing in on what you can and ought to eat. As a matter of fact, research has shown that adding specific food varieties to your eating regimen is pretty much as significant as scaling back others.

The following are seven modern dietary techniques pointed toward diminishing your gambling factors and upgrading your well-being:

1. Pick Fat Calories Shrewdly

Research has uncovered that the aggregate amount of fat you eat truly isn't connected to coronary illness; it's the type of fat you consume that has the best impact. Two unfortunate fats, including saturated and trans fats, raise blood cholesterol and increase the risk of cardiovascular sickness. Be that as it may, two totally different sorts of fat—monounsaturated and polyunsaturated fats—do the polar opposite. Allude to the table underneath to assist with lessening the fat in your eating regimen.

Soaked Fats

Consuming fewer calories high in soaked fats raises "terrible" cholesterol and low-thickness lipoprotein (LDL) and increases the risk of creating atherosclerosis (the restricting of courses brought about by plaque that can prompt a cardiovascular failure or stroke). Soaked fats are by and large strong or waxy at room temperature and are tracked down principally in creature items and tropical oils. Recorded underneath are a few food sources that are high in saturated fat.

Hamburger, pork, sheep, veal, and the skin of poultry
Wieners, bacon, and high-fat lunch-meeting meats (like salami and bologna)
High-fat dairy items, (for example, entire milk, 2% milk, 4% curds)
Margarine and grease
Sauces and flavors produced using creature fat
Most broiled food varieties and quick food varieties
Bacon fat
Tropical oils - palm, palm part and coconut
Treats and desserts made with grease, margarine, or tropical oils

To cut the soaked fat in your eating regimen, make the accompanying replacements:

Rather of... Choose...
Butter   Trans fat-free tub margarine
Customary cheese   Low-fat or nonfat cheddar
Flavor or half and half Nonfat half and half or nonfat creamer
Entire or 2% milk   1% or nonfat (skim) milk
Customary cream cheese   Reduced fat or nonfat cream cheddar
Customary ice cream Nonfat or low-fat frozen yogurt or sorbet
2-4% milk fat cabin cheese   1% or nonfat curds
Alfredo, cream sauces Marinara, primavera, or light olive-oil-based sauces
Customary mayonnaise   Light or nonfat mayonnaise
Prime grades of beef Choice or Select grades of meat

Spareribs   Tenderloin
Chicken with skin on   Chicken without skin
Entire egg Egg whites or egg substitutes
Most food varieties you pick ought to contain something like 2 grams (g) of soaked fat per serving. Something like 7% of your everyday calorie admission ought to come from immersed fats. Contingent upon your calorie level, your day-to-day soaked fat cutoff will change.

Day to day Calories	Daily Soaked Fat Breaking point (g)
1,200	9
1,400	11
1,600	12
1,800	14
2,000	16
2,200	17
2,400	19

Peruse the Sustenance Realities Board on food names

For a food to be marked "trans-fat-free," it should contain something like 0.5 grams of trans fat per serving. Margarine that is to be trans-fat-free ought to contain water or fluid vegetable oil as the primary fixing. These margarines might in any case contain some hydrogenated oil, yet the sum per serving is immaterial. In any case, segment control is critical - when you surpass the serving size, the item is presently not liberated from trans fat.

Trans Unsaturated fats
Trans unsaturated fats raise the "terrible" cholesterol (LDL) and lower the "upside" cholesterol, high-thickness lipoprotein (HDL). Trans unsaturated fats are framed when a fluid fat is switched over completely to strong fat through an interaction called hydrogenation. Numerous makers utilize hydrogenated fats in their fixings since it makes an item with a drawn-out time span

of usability and further developed consistency.

As protected degrees of trans fat to consume every day, so attempt to keep your day-to-day admission as low as could be expected.

Despite the fact that trans unsaturated fats have been to a great extent disposed of from many handled food varieties, they are still in certain food varieties. Here are far to distinguish trans fats.

Any food that contains to some extent hydrogenated oils, (for example, most handled food sources including treats, saltines, seared snacks, and prepared merchandise) will contain some degree of trans fat, regardless of whether the mark states "trans-fat-free." (See box above.) Since the fixings recorded on a food mark are arranged by weight, food sources that contain to some degree hydrogenated oils at the highest point of the fixings list contain more trans fat than those that contain to some degree hydrogenated oils lower on the rundown. In this manner, watch your part size.

Margarine: Stick margarine contains more hydrogenated oil (trans fat) than tub margarine does; while tub margarine contains more hydrogenated oil than fluid margarine. Search for margarine that doesn't contain "to some extent hydrogenated oil" in the fixing list. An example fixing list is incorporated underneath.

Shortening is an illustration of trans fat in its most perfect structure. A few shortenings presently guarantee to be liberated from trans fat; be that as it may, this may just apply to a food's serving size (recall it can in any case have 1/2 gram or less of trans fat per serving.) Tragically the fat presently used to substitute the trans fat in shortening is high in immersed fat, so it's as yet not a solid decision.

Practically all quick food sources and seared food varieties are presently high in trans fat. Some eatery networks, for example, Ruby Tuesday's, presently utilize a non-hydrogenated or trans-fat-free oil to sear their food sources. Yet, recall that a heart-accommodating eating routine contains next to no seared food.

Search for food sources that are named trans-fat-free or those that utilize fluid vegetable oils rather than hydrogenated oils in the fixing list.

Unsaturated Fats

Unsaturated fats are viewed as the best fats since they further develop cholesterol, are related to lower irritation (a gamble factor for coronary illness), and are related to in general lower hazard of creating coronary illness. Unsaturated fats are found fundamentally in plant-based food sources; what's more, are for the most part fluid at room temperature. Unsaturated fat comes in two varieties:

monounsaturated
polyunsaturated
Monounsaturated Fats
Considered quite possibly the best fat source in the eating regimen, monounsaturated fats ought to make up the heft of your everyday fat admission. Monounsaturated fats are tracked down in high focus in these food sources:

Olive oil
Canola (rapeseed) oil
Nut oils
Generally, nuts (barring pecans), nut oils, and nut spreads (like peanut butter)
Olives
Avocados

Polyunsaturated Fats

Polyunsaturated fats are seen as fundamentally in:

Corn oil
Soybean oil
Safflower oil
Flax oil and flax seeds
Sunflower oil
Pecans
Fish
Omega-3 is one kind of poly-unsaturated fat that has extra defensive advantages against cardiovascular illness, including bringing down fatty oils, safeguarding against sporadic pulses, diminishing the gamble of a coronary episode, and bringing down circulatory strain.

Great food wellsprings of omega-3 are fish - particularly cool water fish like mackerel, salmon, herring, and sardines. More modest measures of this defensive fat can likewise be tracked down in flaxseeds, chia seeds (frequently sold as salvia), pecans, soybeans, and canola oils.

To receive the defensive rewards of omega-3 fat, integrate fish into no less than two dinners each week and add plant-based wellsprings of omega-3, like ground flaxseeds and pecans, into your everyday eating plans.

For more data about omega-3 fats, kindly request your dietitian for a duplicate from the freebee, "The Force of Fish: Omega-3 Unsaturated fats."

Cholesterol Decreases and that's just the beginning
Late exploration discoveries show that when unsaturated fats are filled in for certain carbs in the eating routine, these great fats diminish unsafe LDL and expand solid HDL cholesterol. Moreover, supplanting a starch-rich eating routine with one rich in unsaturated fat, fundamentally

monounsaturated, brought down cholesterol as well as circulatory strain and generally speaking coronary illness risk.

All out Fat

As indicated by the most recent public cholesterol rules, your absolute day-to-day fat admission ought to go from 20 to 35 percent of your all-out everyday calories. How much fat you ought to eat relies on your individual cardiovascular infection hazard and lipid levels. Ask your doctor or dietitian for more data.

Your absolute everyday fat ought to come from these sources every day:

Fat Source Recommendation
Monounsaturated Fat 10   to   20%   of everyday calories
Polyunsaturated Fat   10%   or   less   of everyday calories

Soaked in addition to Trans Fat   7%   or less of day-to-day calories

By picking unsaturated fats rather than soaked fats whenever the situation allows, you'll have the option to meet these rules.

2. Limit Dietary Cholesterol

Since cholesterol is produced using the liver, it is just tracked down in food sources of creatures (not in plant-based food sources). For a great many people, how much cholesterol in the eating routine unobtrusively affects their blood cholesterol levels? Be that as it may, there are many individuals whose blood cholesterol levels change firmly with how much cholesterol is eaten. What's more, cholesterol in the eating regimen enormously influences individuals who have diabetes.

Everybody should really try to restrict all dietary cholesterol. Assuming that you have elevated cholesterol, limit your everyday dietary cholesterol to 200 milligrams; in the event that you have ordinary cholesterol levels, break point to 300 milligrams day to day.

Everyday Cholesterol Proposal
Assuming you have elevated cholesterol levels of 200 mg or lower
Assuming you have typical cholesterol levels of 300 mg or lower
The following are a couple of tips to cut cholesterol in the eating routine:

Eat three or less egg yolks each week. Pick egg whites or egg substitutes all things being equal.
Eliminate skin from poultry prior to eating; cut back excess from red meat prior to eating.
Limit red meat and poultry parts to an a3-ounce segment (the size of a deck of cards).
Pick nonfat or low-fat cheeses. Limit absolute cheddar admission to three dinners week by week.

Attempt soy-put-together cheddar choices with respect to sandwiches or meals.

Pick stock over cream-based soups.

Limit high-fat dairy food sources, for example, cream cheddar, 4% curds, or entire milk yogurt; pick nonfat or low-fat assortments.

3. Get Your Everyday Fiber Lift

As a component of a solid eating routine, fiber can lessen cholesterol. Dietary fiber is a kind of carb that the body can't process. It's tracked down principally in entire grains, natural products, vegetables, and beans. As fiber goes through the body, it influences the manner in which the body digests food varieties and retains supplements.

An eating regimen rich in fiber has medical advances past cholesterol control: it assists control of blood sugar, advances consistency, forestalls gastrointestinal illness, and helps in weight the board.

Day to day Fiber Recommendation Age Gathering

38 grams   Men 50 and under

25 grams   Women 50 and under

30 grams   Men more than 50

21 grams   Women more than 50

There are two kinds of dietary fiber: dissolvable and insoluble. Each remarkably affects well-being.

Solvent (thick) fiber: Gives the best heart-medical advantage since it assists with bringing down aggregate and LDL cholesterol. Great wellsprings of solvent fiber incorporate oats, oat grain, grain, vegetables (like dried beans, lentils, and split peas), psyllium, flaxseed, apples, pears, and citrus natural products.

Insoluble fiber: For the most part alluded to as "roughage." Insoluble fiber advances consistency, adds mass and non-abrasiveness to stools, assists with weight guidelines, and forestalls numerous gastrointestinal issues. Great wellsprings of insoluble fiber incorporate wheat, entire wheat, and other entire-grain oats and bread, nuts, and vegetables.

Food varieties contain a blend of dissolvable and insoluble fiber. To get the best medical advantage, eat a wide assortment of high-fiber food sources.

The most effective method to get more fiber in your eating regimen:

Get the day going right with entire-grain cereal or entire-grain toast (in the event that your cholesterol is high, pick oats or oat wheat cereal or toast).
Rather than natural product juice, have an entire piece of organic product.
For a fiber-stuffed lunch, prepare ½ cup garbanzo beans into a verdant green serving of mixed greens.
Pick entire grain buns, bagels, English biscuits, wafers, and bread rather than improved or white assortments.

Buy entire wheat pasta and earthy-colored rice rather than improved assortments.

Top yogurt or curds with new natural products or nuts.

Give zing to stock soup by adding vegetables, dried beans, or grain.

Nibble on new natural products, vegetables, or a hand-crafted nut and dried organic product blend.

Best wellsprings of dietary fiber

The best wellsprings of dietary fiber are crude or cooked foods grown from the ground, entire grain items, and vegetables (like dried beans, lentils, or split peas). Refined food varieties, for example, white bread, pasta, and enhanced grains are low in dietary fiber. The refining system strips the external coat (called the wheat) from the grain, bringing down the fiber content.

Fiber's job in weigh the executives

Subbing enhanced, white pasta and rice and other refined food varieties with entire grain assortments is an incredible method for supporting dietary fiber admission and assisting with forestalling glucose vacillations over the course of the day. This, thus, helps keep you feeling fulfilled and can assist with forestalling unexpected desires for desserts or other fast sugar food sources later in the day. The outcome: weight control.

Understanding the Fiber Content in Food Varieties

High Density At least 5 grams of fiber per serving

(The food should likewise meet the definition for low-fat, or the degree of absolute fat should show up close to the high-fiber guarantee)
A great wellspring of fiber   2.5 g to 4.9 g of fiber per serving

More or added fiber   At least 2.5 g more fiber per serving than the practically identical item
4. Increment Organic products, Vegetables, Vegetables and Nuts

Just three percent of Americans consume the suggested measure of organic products, vegetables, vegetables, and grains suggested by well-being experts. To amplify your admission of coronary illness battling cancer prevention agents, nutrients, minerals, protein, and dietary fiber, embrace the accompanying three systems.

a. Pick 7-A-Day:

Hold back nothing 7 servings of products of the soil (at least) every day. One serving of organic product incorporates:

1 medium-sized piece of new organic product
product
1/2 medium banana

1/2 grapefruit

2 Tbsp dried natural product

1/2 cup canned natural product

1/2 to 3/4 cup most squeezes

One serving of vegetables incorporates:

1/2 cup cooked vegetables

1 cup crude or verdant vegetables

b. Hold back nothing/cup of vegetables no less than multiple times week by week.

Add beans to servings of mixed greens, have parted pea soup, or throw lentils into a rice dish. Vegetables are a force to be reckoned with of defensive supplements - including potassium, fiber, protein, iron, and the B-nutrients.

c. Appreciate 5 ounces of nuts every week.

Specialists have connected normal admission of nuts to a lower frequency of coronary illness. Moderate utilization (something like 1 ounce) of nuts each day furnishes you with numerous defensive supplements like vitamin E, zinc, iron, protein, monounsaturated fats, and dietary fiber. Pick new or dry simmered, unsalted nuts and regular peanut butter for the greatest heart assurance. Keep away from sugar, salted, or oil-broiled assortments. Buy nuts in the mass food segment of the supermarket or close to the baking aisle.

More tips to build natural products, vegetables, and vegetables:

Pack crude vegetables or leafy foods to work for a fast bite.
Purchase pre-sliced vegetables to save time.
Prepare nuts into servings of mixed greens, in sautés or trail blends, or eat them plain.
Spread peanut butter on saltines, celery, toast or even mix into your morning cereal.
Have a vegetable-based soup with your standard sandwich at lunch.
Rather than a treat, partake in a new, fresh apple for dessert.

Keep new natural products directly in front of you or the work area.

Keep dried natural products, nuts, or canned organic products with you in the event that you foresee you'll be feeling the loss of a feast.

5. Substitute Plant Protein for Creature Protein

Increment plant wellsprings of protein and begin lessening your admission of creature protein. Research shows this can really affect heart wellbeing. Subbing non-meat wellsprings of protein for meat fundamentally decreases soaked fat and cholesterol and lifts coronary illness battling fiber, nutrients, minerals, and cancer prevention agents.

Pick 2 to 3 vegetable protein feasts week after week, for example, split pea soup, garbanzo bean salad, soy or dark bean burgers, tofu pan sear, or finished vegetable protein.

Limit red meat admission to something like one feast week by week (this incorporates hamburger, pork, and veal).

Pick 2 skinless poultry feasts week by week.

Hold back nothing of 6 ounces of omega-3-rich fish (two dinners) week by week.

6. Disperse Dinners and Bites

It isn't prescribed to Skip feasts. Little, incessant dinners and tidbits seem to advance weight reduction and upkeep and offer you a chance to consume significant supplements over the course of the day. Skipping feasts just brings down digestion and denies you key supplements. Scientists have found that individuals who balance their calories into four to six little feasts every day have lower cholesterol levels.

This is the way to disseminate feasts and snacks in a heart-accommodating style:

Partition calories into 4 to 6 more modest feasts.

Eat the heft of the day's calories during light hours for the greatest energy.

See the test menu beneath.

Test Little, Successive Dinner Plan

7:00 am - 1 cup cooked cereal with 2 Tbsp raisins, 6 almonds, 8 ounces skim milk.

9:30 am - ½ cup 1% fat, calcium-braced curds blended in with ½ cup canned mandarin oranges (in additional light syrup), 8 ounces of water.

12:15 pm - 2 cups salad (spinach, Romaine, celery, cherry tomatoes, cucumber, carrots, onion, garlic) finished off with ½ cup garbanzo beans and combination of 1 tsp olive oil, 2 Tbsp red wine vinegar; medium apple; 5 entire wheat wafers and 16 ounces water.

3:00 pm - 1 ½ cups crude vegetable blend (green peppers, cauliflower, cherry tomatoes, carrots) dunked in ¼ cup hummus, 8 ounces of water.

6:00 pm - 4 ounces barbecued salmon presented with 1 cup earthy colored rice, 1 ½ cups steamed broccoli, 1 little rye roll with 1 tsp trans-free margarine, and 16-ounce water.

8:00 pm - (discretionary) ½ cup nonfat chocolate pudding finished off with ½ banana, 8 ounces water.

Supplement Investigation: 1,850 calories, 24% complete fat (52 grams), 4% soaked fat (8 grams), 11% monounsaturated fat (19 grams), 5% polyunsaturated fat (10 grams), 95 milligrams cholesterol, 41 grams absolute fiber, 2,200 milligrams sodium.

7. Practice Piece Control

At the point when you are attempting to follow an eating plan that is great for you, it might assist with knowing the amount of a particular sort of food that is thought of as a "serving."; The table beneath offers a few models.

Food/Amount   Serving Size
Reference Size

1 cup cooked pasta or rice   2 starch   Tennis ball

1 cut bread 1 starch   Compact plate case

1 cup crude vegetables or fruit   1 vegetable or fruit Baseball

½ cup cooked vegetables or fruit   1 vegetable or fruit Ice cream scoop

1 ounce low-fat cheese 1 medium-fat protein   Pair of dice

1 teaspoon olive oil   1 fat   Half-dollar

3 ounces cooked meat 3 protein   Deck   of cards or tape

3 ounces tofu   1 protein   Deck of cards or tape

CHAPTER 7

The Role Of Genetics In Blood Disorders

The principal sorts of hereditary blood issues are thalassemia and sickle cell pallor. These problems are passed down from parent to kid through the qualities carried on the chromosomes. At the point when the two guardians have a hereditary deformity, there's a 25% opportunity that every kid will be brought into the world with the sickness.

Hereditary Blood Problems Hereditary blood issues are sent from guardians to their youngsters. Certain blood problems are brought about by the decreased creation of red platelets. Red platelets in our body don't endure forever and are required to have been created after some time, when the development of these red platelets stops it causes blood issues in the body of the people and may result in

some serious illness. There are a few related strange hemoglobin sicknesses, like sickle cell pallor and thalassemia.

Such illnesses can be communicated from guardians to youngsters by qualities on chromosomes. At the point when the two guardians have the sickle cell characteristic, there is a 25% opportunity that a youngster will have sickle cell infection. Yet, when one parent is conveying the characteristic and the other really has the sickness, the chances increase to half that their youngster will acquire the illness.

Spread of Hereditary Blood Issues in the Realm:

The spread of hereditary blood problems (sickle cell weakness and thalassemia) contrasts among the different locales of the Realm. The most elevated rates are tracked down in the eastern and southern districts, while the rates are low in focal and northern locales of the Realm. As per the measurements delivered by the Service of Wellbeing (Wellbeing Marriage Against Hereditary Blood Problems Program: Sickle Cell Sickliness and Thalassemia), from 1425H till the finish of 1430H, the occurrence of sickle cell frailty frequency recorded was 0.27%, while the rate of thalassemia was 0.05%.

What is Sickle Cell Paleness?
Sickle cell pallor is an acquired type of paleness — a condition wherein there aren't sufficient sound red platelets to convey satisfactory oxygen all through your body. Ordinarily, your red platelets are adaptable and round, moving effectively through your veins. In sickle cell frailty, the red platelets become unbending and tacky and are formed like sickles or bow moons. These unpredictably formed cells can stall out in little veins, which can slow or impede blood stream and oxygen to parts of the body.

Side effects of Sickle Cell Pallor

Occasional episodes of agony in various pieces of the body as per the spot for breaking red platelets and microvascular hindrance like torment in mid-region, joints, or one of the gatherings.
 Ongoing iron deficiency.
 Regular diseases.
 Side effects of hunger, short height, and slow development.
 Bone deformations.
 Laziness and weariness.
Entanglements of Sickle Cell Paleness
Entanglements happen because of blockage of little veins and the breakdown of red platelets, and these inconveniences include:
 Coronary failure and stroke.
 Expanded diseases.
 Jaundice is frequently seen by yellowing of eyes and skin.
 Gallstones

Crumbling of the retina because of the absence of sustenance. Harm can prompt fractional or complete visual deficiency

Postpone inappropriate development and accomplishing adolescence in kids. In grown-ups, hindered development or a slow course of development.

Medicines and Medications:

Therapy for sickle cell pallor is generally aimed toward staying away from emergencies, alleviating torment, forestalling entanglements, and working on the capacity of the patient to live with the illness.

Sickle cell paleness patients need ceaseless consideration to forestall a repeat of intricacies and weakening of their well-being status.

Folic corrosive enhancements are suggested to create red platelets.

To ease torment during a sickle emergency the patient is treated with torment prescriptions and expanding liquid admission.

Now and again, the aggravation might answer over-the-counter (OTC) torment prescriptions, while others require more grounded impacts, like morphine and meperidine under clinical watch at emergency clinics.

Treatment with hydroxyurea may decrease the recurrence of excruciating emergencies and of intense chest disorders for grown-ups.

Anti-infection agents are regularly given to forestall diseases in youngsters. Kids and grown-ups ought to get all suggested immunizations, including yearly influenza shots.

Patients don't require blood bondings consistently, as well as in crisis emergencies.

The patient's eyes might be impacted, which can prompt incomplete or complete visual impairment, thus, the patient should be mindful so as to visit an eye specialist consistently.

 Bone marrow transfers can fix sickle cell illness.

What is Thalassemia?

Thalassemia, otherwise called Mediterranean paleness, is a problem that makes the blood contain deficient amounts of red platelets and hemoglobin. This condition is acquired and is most prevalent in people of Italian, Central Asian, Greek, African, Chinese, Filipino, and Southern Asian descent.

Thalassemia Types and Side Effects:

1. Alpha Thalassemia

Alpha thalassemia happens when at least one of the four alpha chain qualities neglects to work. Alpha chain protein creation, for down-to-earth objects, is equitably split between the four qualities. With alpha thalassemia, the "fizzled" qualities are perpetually lost from the cell because of a hereditary mishap.

a) The deficiency of one quality lessens the development of the alpha protein just somewhat. This condition is so near ordinary that it very well may be recognized exclusively by specific lab procedures that, as of not long ago, were restricted to investigate labs. An individual with this condition is known as a "quiet transporter" due to the trouble in identification.

b) The deficiency of two qualities (two-quality cancellation alpha thalassemia) delivers a condition with little red platelets, and probably a gentle sickliness. Individuals with this condition look and feel typical. The condition can be distinguished by routine blood testing, notwithstanding.

c) The deficiency of three alpha qualities delivers a serious hematological issue (three-quality erasure alpha-thalassemia). Patients with this condition have an extreme paleness and frequently require blood bondings to make due. The serious irregularity between the alpha chain creation and beta chain creation (which is ordinary) causes a gathering of beta chains inside the red platelets. Typically, beta chains pair just with alpha chains. With three-quality cancellation alpha thalassemia, notwithstanding, beta chains start to relate in gatherings of four, delivering an unusual hemoglobin, called "hemoglobin H". The condition is designated "hemoglobin H infection".

Hemoglobin H has two issues. First, it doesn't convey oxygen appropriately, making it practically useless to the phone. Second, the hemoglobin H protein harms the layer that encompasses the red cell, speeding up cell obliteration. The mix of the exceptionally low creation of alpha chains and obliteration of red cells in hemoglobin

H sickness delivers an extreme, dangerous sickness. Untreated, most patients bite the dust in youth or early pre-adulthood.

d) The deficiency of every one of the four alpha qualities creates a condition that is inconsistent with life. The gamma chains created during fetal life partner in gatherings of four to shape a strange hemoglobin called "Hemoglobin Barts '. A great many people with four-quality cancellation alpha thalassemia pass on in utero or soon after birth. Once in a while, four quality erasure alpha thalassemia has been distinguished in utero, as a rule in a family where the issue happened in a previous kid. In utero blood bondings have saved a portion of these youngsters. These patients require long-lasting bonding and other clinical help.

2. Beta Thalassemia

Beta thalassemia happens when the beta globin chains are either delivered insufficiently or not in any way shape or form. An individual experiences beta thalassemia when he acquires one deserted beta globin chain from each parent.

There are two kinds of beta thalassemia: major and minor:

Beta thalassemia minor happens when only one of the beta chains is absconded. This outcome results in low degrees of hemoglobin creation in the blood. It affects the body as that of gentle sickness brought about by a lack of iron; albeit the degrees of iron in the blood seem typical.

Thalassemia major, additionally called Cooley's iron deficiency, happens when both beta chains are absconded, which brings about no development of hemoglobin. Beta thalassemia major is a serious perilous condition.

Complications:
Patients with significant thalassemia and hemoglobin H illness experience the ill effects of numerous difficulties in the event that not treated as expected and in an opportune

way, for example,

 Defer in appropriate development.
 Developed spleen, enlarged stomach.
 Bone deformations
  Expanding side effects of sickliness and feeling steady pressure and exhaustion.
 Medicines and Medications

  Patients with significant thalassemia and hemoglobin H sickness necessitates ordinary and constant consideration to forestall the different entanglements of thalassemia, for example, repetitive diseases and crumbling of well-being status, which might prompt demise on the off chance that are not treated as expected.

Contingent upon the seriousness, thalassemia patients go through red platelet bondings.

Folic corrosive enhancements are suggested to create red platelets.

Chelation treatment, ordinarily with the iron-restricting specialist, desferrioxamine (Desferal), is expected to keep demise from iron-intervened organ injury.

Evacuation of the spleen is now and then required.

Bone marrow transfers can help patients who are analyzed right on time before inconveniences.

Anticipation of Hereditary Blood Illnesses:

The obligation to an early assessment assists with lessening the transmission of hereditary blood illnesses across ages; as clinical trials show the conceivable presence of tainted qualities among ladies or men, who don't show side effects.

Around 70,000 to 100,000 Americans have sickle cell illness, the most widely recognized type of an acquired blood problem. This sickness, which is available in impacted people upon entering the world, causes the development of strange hemoglobin.

CHAPTER 8

Supportive Care And Quality Of Life For Individuals With Blood Disorders

Strong consideration assumes a significant part in the treatment of many individuals living with blood conditions. This includes bending over backward to work on your satisfaction, by alleviating any side effects you could have and by forestalling and treating any complexities that emerge from your infection or treatment.

Clinical strong consideration

Blood bondings, antitoxins, intravenous liquids, and comparative therapies, can be in every way significant components of clinical steady consideration. Diseases are a typical intricacy of blood conditions and their medicines which can happen for various reasons, and it is critical to play it safe where conceivable.

Non-clinical steady consideration

Non-clinical strong considerations might include corresponding treatments, sustenance support, exercise, directing, and comparable administrations. Illuminate your hematologist assuming any medical procedure or therapy is arranged by another professional, as counsel might be expected from your hematologist regarding the best strong therapy, for example, bondings, blood tests, or other observing, to guarantee that your therapy happens effectively without issues because of your sickness, current or past therapy.

Backing to continue on

On account of advances in the therapy of blood malignant growths, an ever-increasing number of individuals are relieved, while numerous others experience significant periods where their illness is taken care of. Look at our video 'This is No joking matter' underneath which frames how to live with a blood malignant growth conclusion.

Survivorship brings its arrangement of difficulties and open doors including monetary contemplations, choices about getting back to work, changing connections at work and home, and laying out continuous encouraging groups of people.

Treatment given to free the side effects of an illness and the treatment's aftereffects is known as steady consideration. The objective of steady consideration is to further develop the patient's satisfaction and to alleviate uneasiness however much as could reasonably be expected. Steady consideration is a significant piece of MDS treatment.

Blood Bondings

Bondings of red platelets can help a few patients by further developing their platelet counts or by easing paleness side effects, for example, windedness, unsteadiness, outrageous weariness, and chest torment. Bonding can assist with easing side effects for a brief time frame, yet more bonding might be required over the long haul. In MDS, 60 to 80 percent of patients have frailty at the hour of determination, and up to 90 percent of patients will require at least one bond throughout their ailment.

Platelet bondings might be utilized in patients with thrombocytopenia (low platelet counts), which can cause side effects, for example, simple swelling or death. Bondings are normally required once a patient's platelet count falls under 10,000/mcL or for intense dying. Aminocaproic corrosive and tranexamic corrosive, antifibrinolytic specialists are suggested for draining episodes that don't answer platelet bonding, and for instances of extreme thrombocytopenia. This medicine works by preventing blood clusters from separating excessively fast.

Iron Chelation Treatment
Iron is tracked down in red platelets. At the point when an individual gets countless red platelet bondings, an excess of iron can develop in the body. This is classified as "iron over-burden," and it can harm indispensable organs over the long run.

Iron chelation treatment utilizes drugs called "chelators," which tie to the abundance of iron and eliminate it from the body. This treatment might be suitable for pallid patients who need successive blood bondings (multiple units of red platelets north of about two months). The most well-known drugs utilized in this treatment incorporate

Deferasirox (Exjade®, Jadenu®)
Deferoxamine mesylate (DFO; Desferal®)
For patients who need regular red platelet bondings, it is suggested that specialists screen serum ferritin (iron) levels and check frequently for indications of organ harm.

Platelet Development Variables
Specialists called "development factors" advance platelet creation in the bone marrow. These specialists are utilized to treat a few patients whose platelet counts show diminished quantities of cells.

Red Platelet Development Elements: Erythropoietin (EPO) is a chemical made in the kidneys. It empowers red platelet creation because of low oxygen levels in the body. A deficiency of EPO can likewise cause frailty.

Erythropoiesis-animating specialists (ESAs) are red platelet development factors that are drug analogs of normal EPO. They are utilized for MDS patients who have iron deficiency related to low EPO levels. Treatment with ESAs might diminish bonding needs and conceivably further develop endurance.

Epoetin alfa (Procrit®) and darbepoetin alfa (Aranesp®) are kinds of ESAs. They are given by an infusion under the skin (subcutaneously [SC]). Darbepoetin alfa is a more drawn-out acting type of EPO than epoetin alfa.
A few MDS patients with low EPO levels may not profit from treatment with ESAs alone; nonetheless, an ESA given alongside G-CSF might expand their hemoglobin fixation (see beneath).

White Platelet Development Variables: White platelet development factors are normally created by the body, and assist with expanding the creation of white platelets. Manufactured forms of these substances might be utilized to treat patients with successive contaminations because of neutropenia, yet they are not known to assist patients with living longer. The two principal types are

The granulocyte state animating element (G-CSF) which assists the body with expanding white platelet creation. Filgrastim (Neupogen®) and Pegfilgrastim (Neulasta®) are instances of G-CSF prescriptions.
Granulocyte-macrophage province animating element (GM CSF) assists the body with delivering various sorts of white platelets. Sargramostim (Leukine®) is a GM CSF prescription.

Platelet Development Elements: Thrombopoietin (TPO) is a substance that assists the body with delivering platelets.

Romiplostim (Nplate®) and eltrombopag (Promacta®) are drugs that carry on like TPO. These specialists are being examined as a treatment for MDS patients who have low platelet counts. Presently, these medications are FDA-supported for the therapy of thrombocytopenia (low platelet counts) in patients who have persistently resistant thrombocytopenic purpura (ITP) and who have had a lacking reaction to corticosteroids, immunoglobulins, or splenectomy.

Even though romiplostim and eltrombopag are not explicitly supported for MDS, some of the time they can be useful in patients with extremely low platelet counts.

Erythroid Development Specialists: Erythroid development specialists are utilized to treat frailty. They work by directing red platelet development.

Luspatercept-amt (Reblozyl®) is FDA-supported for the treatment of:

Iron deficiency without past erythropoiesis animating specialist use (ESA-guileless) in grown-up patients with exceptionally low-to-middle-of-the-road risk myelodysplastic disorders (MDS) who might require standard red platelet (RBC) bondings.

Paleness bombing an erythropoiesis animating specialist and requiring at least 2 RBC units north of about two months in grown-up patients with exceptionally low-to-middle gamble myelodysplastic disorders with ring sideroblasts

Constraints of Purpose: Reblozyl isn't demonstrated for use as a substitute for RBC bondings in patients who require prompt remedy of pallor.

CONCLUSION

In conclusion, finding solutions to blood disorders is an important step toward improving the quality of life for millions of people all over the world. As we dig into the complex idea of these problems, it turns out to be progressively obvious that an extensive methodology is important to address the different scope of conditions included by the expression "blood problems." Through logical progressions, clinical developments, and an all-encompassing comprehension of the mind-boggling systems overseeing blood well-being, a promising scene unfolds, offering expectations for both current and future generations.

One of the critical parts of the answer to blood problems lies in hereditary examination and customized medication. With the interpretation of the human genome, scientists have acquired extraordinary experiences in the hereditary premise of different blood problems. This information has been prepared for designated treatments, permitting medical services experts to tailor therapy plans in light of a person's hereditary cosmetics. Customized medication improves treatment viability as well as limits unfriendly impacts, denoting a change in perspective in the way we approach and oversee blood problems.

In addition, research into stem cells emerges as a sign of hope in the search for treatments for blood disorders. Immature microorganisms, with their momentous capacity to separate into different cell types, hold gigantic potential for regenerative medication. Researchers are investigating the utilization of foundational microorganisms to supplant harmed or broken platelets, offering a notable way to deal with conditions like iron deficiency, leukemia, and different issues influencing the blood and bone marrow. The commitment to undeveloped cell treatments stretches out the simple side effects of the board, indicating the chance of long haul and, surprisingly, remedial interventions.

The job of innovation in blood jumble arrangements couldn't possibly be more significant. State-of-the-art advances like CRISPR-Cas9 quality altering hold monstrous commitment in revising hereditary peculiarities answerable for specific blood issues. The accuracy and productivity of CRISPR-Cas9 open up new roads for restorative interventions, possibly permitting researchers to alter illness-causing changes at the hereditary level. While moral contemplations and security concerns remain, the capability of quality-altering advancements to upset the treatment scene for blood problems is unquestionable.

Schooling and mindfulness play a pivotal role in the more extensive treatment of blood problems. The public's awareness of the importance of regular blood screenings, early detection, and preventative measures can significantly reduce the burden of these disorders. Outfitting medical services experts with exceptional information and assets guarantees that people get convenient and accurate conclusions, encouraging a proactive instead of responsive way to deal with the blood jumble of the executives.

A joint effort between specialists, medical service suppliers, drug organizations, and policymakers is fundamental in the quest toward powerful answers for blood problems. A deliberate effort to share information, pool assets, and smooth out administrative cycles can speed up the turn of events and the spread of creative treatments. Worldwide joint efforts, specifically, can work with the sharing of different points of view, assets, and skills, making a synergistic impact that rises above topographical limits while chasing compelling arrangements.

All in all, the answer to blood problems is a dynamic and developing embroidery woven together by headways in hereditary qualities, regenerative medication, innovation, training, and joint effort. As we disentangle the intricacies of these issues, the aggregate endeavors of mainstream researchers, medical care experts, and policymakers meet to offer a more promising time to come for those impacted. Through a thorough and interdisciplinary methodology, we stand at the limit of a groundbreaking leap forward that holds the possibility to lighten the suffering of people wrestling with blood issues and usher in another time of well-being and prosperity.

9 798878 552561